Ultimate Mindful Eating Guide!

Mindful Eating

Stop Overeating And Binge Eating For Good And Lose Weight With Mindfulness, Self Discipline, Meditation, And Willpower Strategies!

I0428320

Sarah Brooks

Copyright © 2014 Sarah Brooks

STOP!!! Before you read any further....Would you like to know the Secrets of Body Transformation?

If your answer is yes, then you are not alone. Thousands of people are looking for the secret to rapidly burn body fat, keep the weight off, become healthier, and truly transform their body and life for good.

If you have been searching for these answers without much luck, you are in the right place!

Not only will you gain incredible insight in this book, but because I want to make sure to give you as much value as possible, right now for a limited time you can get full **100% FREE access to a VIP bonus EBook** entitled **THE 7 KEYS TO BODY TRANSFORMATION!**

Just Go Here For Free Instant Access:

www.liveFitVIP.com

Legal Notice

All rights reserved. Without limiting the rights under the copyright reserved above, no part of this publication may be reproduced, stored in or introduced into a retrieval system, or transmitted, in any form, or by any means (electronic, mechanical, photocopying, recording, or otherwise) without the prior written permission of the copyright owner and publisher of this book. This book is copyright protected. This is for your personal use only. You cannot amend, distribute, sell, use, quote or paraphrase any part or the content within this eBook without the consent of the author or copyright owner. Legal action will be pursued if this is breached.

Disclaimer Notice

Please note the information contained within this document is for educational and entertainment purposes only. Considerable energy and every attempt has been made to provide the most up to date, accurate, relative, reliable, and complete information, but the reader is strongly encouraged to seek professional advice prior to using any of this information contained in this book. The reader understands they are reading and using this information contained herein at their own risk, and in no way will the author, publisher, or any affiliates be held responsible for any damages whatsoever. No warranties of any kind are expressed or implied. Readers acknowledge that the author is not engaging in the rendering of legal, financial, medical, or any other professional advice. By reading this document, the reader agrees that under no circumstances is the author, publisher, or anyone else affiliated with the production, distribution, sale, or any other element of this book responsible for any losses, direct or indirect, which are incurred as a result of the use of information contained within this document, including, but not limited to, -errors, omissions, or inaccuracies. Because of the rate with which conditions change, the author and publisher reserve the right to alter and update the information contained herein on the new conditions whenever they see applicable.

Table Of Contents

Introduction

I want to thank you and congratulate you for purchasing the book, *"Mindful Eating: Ultimate Mindful Eating Guide! - Stop Overeating And Binge Eating For Good And Lose Weight With Mindfulness, Self Discipline, Meditation, And Willpower Strategies!"*

This Mindfulness Eating book contains proven steps and strategies on how to avoid overeating and binge eating for good. It is easy to fall into the trap of mindless eating especially given the world's culture today, but it does not mean that overeating should be a normal part of life.

Overeating and binge eating can lead to serious health problems and issues, and it is time that people take an active stance against such issues. Lead a healthy and well-balanced life by following simple steps and strategies that will keep you off your cravings and away from binge eating.

Thanks again for purchasing this book, I hope you enjoy it!

Chapter 1: What Does Mindful Eating Mean? What Does Binge Eating Mean?

Eating is a natural way of life. People, along with all the other animals and living things in the world need to eat or consume foods in order to grow and survive. However, there is more to eating than simply shoving up food into our mouths.

Mindful Eating

In the world today where food seems to be everywhere, the act of eating becomes what is known as a mindless deed. There is hardly any thought that goes along with the action and many people seem to just eat whatever food is right before them. In some cases, people are not even aware of the foods that they consume or would simply forget about them mere minutes after they have eaten. These facts tell us that the act of mindless eating is so rampant that it oftentimes leads to guilt and weight and health related problems. If there is such a thing as mindless eating, what is mindful eating then?

To some, mindful eating is the act of being fully aware of and in control of what they eat. This means that they pay every attention to the foods they eat and are therefore able to notice and enjoy every bite they take. It also means being aware of the foods' effects on the body, and therefore having the intention of taking care of oneself. After all, no one would mindfully eat something if there is a known negative effect on the self. To this respect, mindful eating builds a peaceful relationship with the body where the body's needs and sometimes even the wants, are satisfied. It becomes an act of wisdom and of full consciousness as it chooses what is natural and healthy.

Binge Eating

On the other end of the spectrum is what is known as binge eating. This is the earlier form of eating that was discussed as being mindless, and even sometimes taken to an extreme level. Binge eating is defined as disordered eating wherein the act is uncontrollable. This leads to eating enormous amounts of food even after the individual has had the feeling of a full stomach.

Most people who suffer from binge eating try to hide it from friends and family, leading them to isolate themselves in many instances.

In extreme cases, binge eating is a serious disorder where one consumes unusually excessive amounts of food. Even those who are not diagnosed with the disorder can experience occasional bouts of binge eating where they find themselves unable to restrain themselves from eating. In some books, the definition of binge eating is excessive and uncontrollable eating that is followed by feelings of guilt and shame. This compulsive eating disorder also leads to many weight and health problems including but not limited to obesity and excessive weight gain. Women have been found to make up 60% of those with binge eating symptoms and one in every five women have reported to experiencing symptoms of binge eating.

Chapter 2: The Top 10 Reasons Why We Overeat

Overeating can lead to weight gain and serious health problems, but most people are guilty of doing it every once in a while. The problem is that overeating is often an unconscious act. Those who do it do not even know that they are overeating. While no one wants to overeat or to simply eat mindlessly, there are reasons why we do so, and they are not as simple as we think. Here are some of the top reasons why people overeat.

Boredom

People eat when they are bored and this happens a lot. One of the main reasons why people overeat is because they have nothing to do, leading them to eating which is the most convenient and easy act. When people are at home and have nothing to do, it is easy for them to open the fridge or grab a snack from the pantry. Even when going outside, eating is one of the most popular activities that people find themselves doing when they want something to do. Eating can be done almost anywhere and at any time of the day, and many people will find that a lot of their time is spent doing so.

Stress and Anxiety

Stress and anxiety are among the top reasons why people overeat. When a person is frustrated or is faced with problems and anxieties, food becomes a default solution. Not that it solves the problem, but eating does give a sense of relief and security.

Coping with Emotions

In relation to coping with stress and anxiety, overeating is also often caused by other strong feelings or emotion. Those who are depressed, for example, find themselves drowning their sorrows in dishes of food. On the other hand, even those who are elated find themselves celebrating over huge servings of food.

For Comfort

The term 'comfort food' is not just something to persuade people to eat. For most people, there is nothing more comforting than a serving or two of their favorite dishes. Eating for comfort is very common as food gives feelings of satiation, well-being, and of course happiness.

Out of Habit

Eating is a part of life and is needed for survival; but most of the time, people eat simply out of habit. While it is just right that we eat on a regular basis, there are times when people eat just because they are used to doing so. People eat after waking up, during all their breaks at school or at work or simply when they find food or when they have nothing else to do. Like the other reasons why people overeat, eating, because of habit, is mindless and not a necessity.

Socialization

Food is almost always at the center of social situations and for this reason, many people find themselves eating more than they should. When out with friends or when celebrating special occasions, food is always sure to be involved. There are also many events where food is part of the equation. Parties always present tables filled with foods, the movies always bring popcorn and snacks, and even the workplace is filled with finger foods, coffee and drinks, or that nearby food chain where employees are sure to spend a lot of their time.

Tired and Deprived

People eat because they are tired and while this only sounds logical, there are times when tiredness leads them to eat even when they are not hungry. Food becomes a pick-me-up tool that helps people get over their tiredness. However, tiredness is not the same as hunger and while food may provide a temporary solution, it can also lead to weight gain and other health problems related to overeating.

Food Everywhere

Overeating is simple to do simply because there is food everywhere. There is food inside the house, food stalls in almost every street and food chains in almost every corner. There are even food vendors who come to you so that you do not even have to look for food yourself. The result is people eat even when they do not need to simply because food is there.

Cravings

Cravings are among the top reasons why people overeat. There are times when people simply feel the need to consume certain types of food. In most cases, we cannot even explain these urges, but they are there. You may crave for a burger or a hot fudge sundae, or a nice big juicy steak. Whatever your craving is, the effect is for you to eat more than you need to and oftentimes, you will eat even more just because you are unable to get what it is you are craving for.

Eating Mindlessly

Eating mindlessly can cause anyone to eat way too much and this is what happens to most of us. The problem is that when people are eating, they are hardly thinking about what they are doing. Instead, their minds are on other things and this leads them to not be aware of how much they are eating. Connected to this is the fact that most people also eat while doing other things. Eating becomes a mindless act that is often done alongside watching TV or while talking with friends and in the end, much more is consumed than if the person is fully aware of what and how much he is eating.

Chapter 3: 5 Simple Steps To Stop Binge Eating Now

There are many things that lead people to eat more than they should, but this does not mean that avoiding overeating is a difficult thing to do. It may be challenging, but being aware of what you are eating and what you are doing is a very fulfilling thing to do, and it also keeps you from doing things that you might later on regret. Stop binge eating by following these 5 simple steps that can help you be healthier today.

1. Eat to satisfy yourself

   Eating is a way of life and is a means for survival, but it should not be taken as a chore or something that is taken for granted. Instead, eat to fulfill your needs and even your wants. Most people take eating for granted or simply something to pass the time. Instead, enjoy what you are eating and therefore, eat what makes you feel good as well. Satisfying yourself also reduces your cravings for more food so you can definitely control the amount you eat.

2. Keep your body active

   There are many instances when people eat simply out of boredom or simply to have anything to do. If this becomes a problem and you find yourself eating too much because of such reasons, then make a change and keep your body active. An active body and lifestyle not only helps you burn those calories, but also keep your mind and your hands away from food. The next time you find yourself looking for something to do, hit the gym, go out for a walk, or simply keep yourself busy with more productive things to do around the house so you do not end up eating more than you should.

3. Learn mindful eating

   Mindless eating is almost synonymous to binge eating and the results is that many people eat foods in amounts that are simply not healthy for them. Instead, be mindful of what you eat and take the time to actually think about what you consume. Do you really want that donut? Are you sure that you need another slice of pizza? Think of what you are eating and know that there are the right foods and the right amounts of food that will keep you satisfied.

4. Fight the urge

It is so hard to say no to urges and cravings but when you learn to do so, you will find that you can actually live without the things that you crave. Urges are often brought on by triggers such as an advertisement perhaps or a friendly suggestion. There are times when the urges are so strong that you will do anything to get what you want, but let a bit of time pass and you will see that the urge or craving will simply pass. Your urge is a fleeting feeling that you can control. Don't give in and keep yourself occupied so that you don't have to surrender to your feelings.

5. Make binge eating inconvenient

Most of us eat because it is easy to do, so stop binge eating by making it inconvenient. Limit the amount of junk food and other ready-to-eat food that you have available at home. If you can, stick to fresh foods that need to be prepared and cooked before you can eat them. The extra time will lessen whatever cravings you have and it will also keep you busy for a longer period of time. When going out, you can also limit your food intake by setting a budget for yourself. Not only do you stop yourself from eating more, but you also get to have a few savings as well.

Chapter 4: 5 Simple Steps To Stop Overeating Now

Binge eating and mindless eating are not the only battles that most people have to face. Along with them is the challenge of overeating. Many people simply eat too much or more than they need. This leads to weight gain, getting fat, and having an unhealthy body. If you want to stop overeating now, try these simple steps.

1. Accept the challenge

   If you want to accomplish anything, you have to first set your mind on it. Accept the fact that you are eating too much and decide to do something about it. Take the challenge to stop overeating, set up your goals, and make sure to be aware of what you want and make sure that everything you do is aligned with them. Stop yourself from overeating by deciding to and by being mindful and aware.

2. Choose health

   The next step that will help you stop overeating is to choose health. Aim to be healthy and make your decisions based on this desire. If you need to eat, choose the healthier options and avoid always eating at fast food chains. Pick out healthy snacks as well such as fruits or even sandwiches instead of going for chips and processed snacks. By deciding to eat healthier, you will find that you will actually be eating just the right mount to keep your body satisfied.

3. Don't let your emotions eat you

   People tend to eat too much when they let their emotions rule them. There are those who overeat because of depression or sorrow, while others eat a lot because of stress and other problems. To stop overeating, never let your emotions rule over your eating habits. This is also related to being mindful of what you eat and how much you eat as you become aware of what it is you do need and what it is that you don't. If you don't need to eat anymore, just stop. Do not make excuses that you are hurt or that you are simply enjoying yourself. If you must, deal with your emotions first and never make them an excuse to eat more or to eat the things that you shouldn't.

4. Manage portion size and pace

Eating too much has much to do with control and sometimes, all it takes is for you to be extra mindful to make sure that you retain that control and that you do not overeat. If you want to avoid eating too much, control your portion sizes and just how fast you eat. For every meal, try to plan out how much protein, starch, and vegetables you should be getting. Get just enough on your plate and avoid taking second servings.

One trick that will help you feel full with less is to simply eat slowly. Chew your food well before swallowing, and take time between bites. This gives your body enough time to send signals that you are already being fed, making you feel satisfied even if you have not eaten much yet. You can also limit the size of your plate. A bigger plate is easier to fill with more food while smaller plates will give you the illusion that you already have much on your plate when you have just enough.

5. Do not deprive yourself

Letting yourself get hungry is almost a sure way to get you to overeat. The hungrier you are, the more your body craves and once you get a taste of food at this point, you will feel the urge to eat even more than you should. Stop overeating by stopping to deprive yourself. This means that you should avoid any fad diets that tell you to eat less and less. In fact, you should eat as often as every three to four hours. Of course, be mindful of choosing healthy options when you do eat. This also means eating at proper times of the day and therefore, this means that you have to fuel yourself every morning with a satisfying breakfast.

Chapter 5: Embracing Mindful Eating And Learning How To Put It In Practice

One of the reasons that lead to binge eating or overeating is forgetting how to eat mindfully. People eat without thinking about what they actually eat, and there are hardly times when one is truly satisfied with the food that they eat. If you practice to do the opposite however and learn to be mindful about what you eat, you will find that you will eat just right and that you will be satisfied even more.

Mindful eating has been described as being fully aware of the food that one eats and of having control over the consumption of such foods. It also means being aware of the effects of those foods on the body, therefore allowing mindfulness to lead to healthy eating as it is only right to consume only those that will benefit the body. To put mindful eating into practice, it is first very important to understand what it is, what it can do for you and how you can make daily decisions that will help you be mindful about what you eat.

Benefits of Mindful Eating

The benefits of mindful eating range farther from physical satisfaction, but it is perhaps one of the most important ones. When people learn to be mindful of what they eat, they gain more pleasure and satisfaction from it. Being mindful means being fully aware of what currently is at the present moment. This means you take in the sight of your food, the delectable aroma and even the different textures that play in your mouth. Most of all, you will take time to savor every taste. In doing so, you will learn to appreciate your food more because you begin to experience it as it truly is. Is it warm and savory? Sweet and velvety? Is there a balance between the flavors present in the dish? All of these things will not only help you enjoy your foods, but will also give your body the feeling of satisfaction.

It is obvious that eating will make you feel full and satisfied, but mindful eating also has the added benefit of letting you eat just right instead of too much. Mindless eating leads people to eat more because they are not aware of how much they eat or whether or not their hunger has already been satisfied. There is also the tendency to eat less healthy foods as you are not fully aware of what you are eating and what its effects are on your body. This is why mindful eating is recommended for eating right and healthy.

Before eating just anything that is being offered, take time to notice what it is that your body really needs and what your food options are. If you are hungry, will you choose a chocolate bar or a filling sandwich? You can go to the nearest fast food chain, or you can take a little more time in enjoying well-cooked foods or natural options. Just because fast food or junk food is there does not mean that they are the only options. Know what your body wants and needs and choose wisely before you eat.

Practice Mindful Eating

Mindful eating aims to change the way people tend to eat without actually thinking of and appreciating what they eat. In order to do this, there are some steps that you can do so that you become more aware not only of the foods you eat, but of their benefits and everything else about them. One of the best things you can do to start practicing mindful eating is to try and cook your own food. Cooking lets you know what goes into your meals and also lets you control what food you can eat. Start out by trying your own favorite dishes at home. By doing so, you will also learn to appreciate your food more and you will also be able to have something to do on your free time.

Once you are comfortable with familiar dishes, you can try experimenting with new dishes as well. There is virtually no limit when you do your cooking by yourself and you can choose to prepare healthier dishes as well. Also, try to experiment with flavor combinations that you like. Cooking will let you appreciate certain foods and will offer unlimited options that can make you change the way you eat.

Mindful eating can also be done even when you are eating outside. Instead of just going for the usual or whatever looks good on the menu, think through your options clearly. What foods are available and what is it that you really want? Giving what your body wants will help satisfy it better. Of course, you should also be mindful of the benefits of the food that you choose. Will it be filling enough? Is it healthy instead of greasy and fatty? Take time to choose well and to choose wisely.

Others who practice mindful eating as a means of dieting will even go so far as understanding about the components of the dish. Where do the ingredients come from and what type of cooking method was used? Locally produced and fresh foods are ideal for processed ingredients while healthier cooking methods such as steaming or grilling are more preferred to frying. You can even ask the restaurant staff about the dishes that they serve and what recommendations they may have. This helps you to know more about what you eat and again, to have a better appreciation of what goes into the food you take.

Finally, practice mindful eating by listening to your body. Understand what foods your body prefers and be aware when your body is full and satisfied. If you eat but do not eat those that are satisfying to the body, you will simply crave what your body wants and therefore eat mindlessly in an attempt to do so. Similarly, if you eat without becoming aware of whether or not your body is already satisfied, you will end up eating more and more and you will not even feel like you have been fed well enough. Appreciation and awareness are the key to mindful eating.

Chapter 6: Self Discipline Strategies To Overcome Cravings And Stop Before You Start Overeating Or Binge Eating

Having concrete ideas and plans will help you to reach your goals better. If your goal is to stop yourself from overeating and binge eating, there are self-discipline strategies that can help you get on the right track.

1. Write down your goal

   It is easy to make up your mind and say that you will stop binge eating and overeating, but it is even easier to forget about such plans and commitments. To make sure that you are reminded of your goals, write them down and place them where you are bound to see them. Right notes such as 'eat healthy' and 'no to junk food' and put them on the refrigerator door or on the pantry shelf. Make simple and daily reminders to help keep your goal in mind so that you make your decisions with such goals in mind.

2. Have some plans

   If you want to reach your goals, you should carry out specific plans and steps that will get you there. For example, plan out your daily or even weekly meals to avoid having to settle for fast food or junk foods. Using the tips mentioned above, write down your menu for breakfast, lunch, dinner, as well as the snacks of the day. Of course, prepare the foods ahead of time so that you will be able to stick to the plan. When going out, plan out activities as well so that you do not end up spending most of the time eating out.

3. Prepare some 'if-then' plans

   Overeating is easily done as a means of coping with emotions or even as a way of spending idle time. Instead of resorting to food as the default option, prepare 'if-then' plans that will keep you away from unnecessary eating. For example, if bored, read a book or go for a walk. If you are tired, play with your pet or listen to some music. Do things that will keep your mind off of food or to simply keep yourself busy. If you do feel the need for snacks, make simple sandwiches or even go for making your own tea or coffee. You should not deprive yourself but food should not be taken for granted either. There are also 'if-then' plans that you can carry out when you have cravings or urges such as going out for a jog or to talk with friends or even simply counting slowly to help let the feeling pass.

4. Avoid eating while doing other things
   Mindless eating is easy to do when you eat without thinking about it. As a strategy to keep yourself from overeating or binge eating, savor every meal and every bite and avoid eating when busy with other things. This includes eating while watching the TV or while playing video games, or even when reading a good book. Doing another thing alongside eating will keep you from being mindful of what you eat and you also fail to be aware of whether or not you are already satisfied. Again, eat for pleasure and to satisfy yourself and savor every dish.

5. Eat slow

   One of the simplest things to do to stop binge eating and to control your cravings is to eat slowly and properly. As explained earlier, taking the time to appreciate your food not only helps you be in control of what you eat but also lets your body adjust more easily. Do you ever notice that you feel full after a certain period of time has elapsed? It will take approximately 15-20 minutes before your body can register that you are feeding it. This means that for the first fifteen minutes, you can virtually feed yourself anything and any amount of food and you will not have any feelings of fullness. Eat slowly and you will find yourself satisfied with less. As for cravings, they are better satisfied if every bite is appreciated.

Chapter 7: How To Build Your Willpower Up And Prepare In Advance For Cravings To Binge Eat

Although the steps and strategies listed above may seem simple in written form, they are actually quite challenging to carry out. To build your willpower up and to prepare yourself against cravings and binge eating, you need the right mindset and attitude. The right mindset is important as it will help you stay focused on what you want, and the right attitude will keep you on the right track no matter what challenges come your way.

Build your willpower by reading about the benefits of mindful eating or even about the negative effects of binge eating. Being more knowledgeable about a certain topic always helps people make up their minds. If knowing about the health benefits is not enough, talk to experts and get sound advice from them. Another way to inform yourself is to talk to other people about it. You may not talk about it but you could actually be facing the same issues with friends or family members. Not only will this give you more information but you will also be able to talk to other people about your concerns.

This is another point that will help you build your willpower up. Establish a support group that you can rely on to help you face your cravings and binge eating issues. Let them know what you are going through and tell them that you are indeed decided on stopping such unhealthy habits. Letting other people know about what you are going through will help them understand your situation more and they will hopefully adjust for you as well.

Instead of enjoying nights out with friends at the nearest fast food store, you can all have a cook fest in one of your homes. You could even make cooking at home a bonding session for the whole family. Of course, having a support group also means you can talk with people if you feel your will is slipping. The most important thing is to know that you are not alone and that the challenge does not have to be a lonely and sad one.

Finally, have some self-confidence. This is another thing that is easier said than done, but the more you instill this in your mind, the easier it is to turn it into reality. Always believe that you can overcome your cravings and your binge eating issues. Instead of becoming fearful of the temptations or triggers that could have you eating too much, believe that you can overcome them.

Of course, it is easier to stay away from temptation during the earlier stages of your endeavor, but you will eventually have to face them. Have your support group with you if you are still doubtful of your own capabilities. Slowly and over time, you will see that the more accomplishments you get, the better your self-confidence will get.

This also leads to another tip: be mindful of and happy about simple accomplishments. If you said no to that slice of pizza, give yourself a pat on the back and congratulate yourself instead of thinking too much about what you missed and regretting it. Having self-confidence is largely a state of mind, but it is also the result of small accomplishments that build character.

This means that you should strive to do things that are in line with your goals. Work out on a regular basis or make a habit of reading about new topics every once in a while. Not only will you be addressing your cravings and binge eating issues but also, you will develop the person that you are.

Chapter 8: Mindfulness Techniques To Enrich Your Mindful Eating Transformation And Enjoy Your Eating Like Never Before

Mindfulness techniques and exercises can help to enrich one's transformation towards mindful eating. These techniques allow a person to appreciate what is in the now so that they may enjoy eating like never before.

- Slow Eating – eating slowly can help a person appreciate food very much. Do this by taking as much time as you can to savor and not just finish a certain type of food. For example, if you have a simple piece of pastry, take the time to enjoy it. Take of the packaging as slowly and as carefully as you can, taking care to keep the pastry as intact as possible. Be sure to note the aroma that comes with opening the package.

  Once you are able to hold it, appreciate the texture as well as the sight. As you take a bite, smell the pastry once again and slowly sink your teeth into it. Let the food rest in your mouth and play with it using your tongue. Enjoy it, savor it and know that you can slowly eat anytime you choose to so that you can appreciate your food more.

- Memory Eating – Food is about taste, satisfaction, and also about memories. When you eat food, what memories does it remind you of? Think back of those times and recall how happy the food has made you. Did the food lighten the situation? Did it help you and your companions feel closer? There are bonds and memories formed over eating, and even these need to be enjoyed and reminisced from time to time.

- Rest Your Hands – Eating is not a laborious process and should be enjoyed while the body is relaxed and satisfied. In order to practice mindful eating, try resting your hands every once in a while. Whether your hands are tired or not, rest your hands after every other bite or so for about 10-20 seconds. This helps you to eat slowly, to get fuller with less, and also to get the time to notice the simple but wonderful aspects of your dish.

Chapter 9: Meditation Strategies To Gain Inner Peace And Gain Better Awareness Of The Food You Eat

Meditation is a practice that increases one's consciousness and when made a habit, can also help to gain better awareness of the foods that one eats. While most meditation techniques are used for relaxation and for building one's values, there are those that can help stop overeating and binge eating.

- Prepare a comfortable space – Meditation is best practiced in a comfortable space where one can relax and truly be in tune with the self. Even when eating, one can practice the meditation strategy of building a comfortable environment by making sure that the table is set well and presentably. Make the dining area neat and remove any unnecessary distractions. Even the arrangement of the plates and the meal itself should be something that is inviting and soothing to all the senses.

- Breathing exercises – Breathing is an integral part of meditation and mindfulness and it helps not only to soothe and relax the body, but also to appreciate every second of every moment. Practice breathing exercises such as deep breaths; and when eating, apply the same techniques so that you do not end up eating too fast and too much. Let your body rest between bites and take the time to appreciate even the simplest details about your dish.

- Remove distractions – Distractions can easily keep one from being conscious of what is happening around them or even of what they themselves are doing. As a meditation strategy to help stop overeating and binge eating, distractions should be removed to help one be mindful of the food that is being eaten. These distractions include the television, mobile phones and tablets, and even books and the newspaper. If you plan on doing other things along with eating, make sure to pause and take time to pay proper attention to each task at hand.

Chapter 10: Simple 5 Minute Daily Routine To Stop Overeating And Binge Eating For Good And To Make Mindful Eating A Lasting Habit

Overeating and binge eating are difficult to stop especially if they have become habits or parts of our lives. Fortunately, there are also habits or daily routines that one can practice to overcome such challenges. This simple 5-minute daily routine will practice mindfulness and meditation that will help to stop overeating and binge eating for good and make mindful eating a lasting habit.

1. Start with a breath – As you sit down at the table, be careful to notice the dishes that are set in front of you. Breathe in then out as you take a moment to take everything in. This allows you to block other distractions and to be aware of the food that you are about to eat.

2. Follow with a prayer – After taking in the food that is before you, take the time to also say a prayer of thanks for what you are about to eat. If you are not the religious type, it does not even have to be a prayer. A simple 'thank you' for the food, and also to the people who made the food possible will be enough to keep you aware of the fact that there is value in what you are about to eat and should therefore not be taken for granted.

3. Sip of water – While not many people do so, starting the meal with a sip of water can help in many ways to stop overeating. For one, drinking water will help make the body feel full faster. Also, drinking water cleanses the palate and helps it become prepared for the food that is about to be eaten. This means that the more water you drink, the fuller you feel and the better you will be able to taste the food that you are eating.

4. Set up your plate – The next thing is for you to set up the food on your plate. Make it as presentable as possible so that you will enjoy it all the more. Try basic plating techniques such as placing the main piece at the side of the plate closest to you and having the sidings at the top. The

better your plate looks, the better you will be able to enjoy it.

5. Enjoy the food – Finally, take your first bite by getting a little bit of everything and placing it on your spoon and finally in your mouth. Getting a little bit of everything will make you enjoy the full flavors of the food. Doing so will also take some time and will help you be aware of all the components of your dish. Place the bits of food in your mouth, bite on it, chew, and let the food run along your tongue. Try to chew as much as you can before swallowing and be mindful of the flavors that course through your tongue.

All of these tasks will take five minutes of your time, sometimes more or sometimes less, but they will definitely take not too much of your time. Most importantly, this simple routine will help you stop overeating and binge eating and will make mindful eating a regular habit.

Conclusion

Eating is a natural way of life and should be a healthy and satisfying act. Stop binge eating and overeating now and lead a healthy life! Also, support your friends and family and help people become aware and mindful of how and what eating should be.

Thank you again for purchasing this book on strategies and steps to stop overeating and binge eating!

I am extremely excited to pass this information along to you, and I am so happy that you now have read and can hopefully implement these strategies going forward.

I hope this book was able to help you understand what mindful eating is and how to practice it in everyday life.

The next step is to get started using this information and to hopefully live a healthy and satisfied life!

Please don't be someone who just reads this information and doesn't apply it, the strategies in this book will only benefit you if you use them!

If you know of anyone else that could benefit from the information presented here please inform them of this book.

Finally, if you enjoyed this book and feel it has added value to your life in any way, please take the time to share your thoughts and post a review on Amazon. It'd be greatly appreciated!

Thank you and good luck!

Preview Of:

Ultimate Superfoods Health And Diet Detox Guide!

<u>Superfoods</u>

Increase Metabolism, Natural Beauty And Health With 50 Powerful Remedies And Recipes For Anti-Aging, Fat Loss, And More!

Introduction

I want to thank you and congratulate you for purchasing the book, *Superfoods: Ultimate Superfoods Health And Diet Detox Guide! - Increase Metabolism, Natural Beauty And Health With 50 Powerful Natural Remedies And Recipes For Anti-Aging, Fat Loss, And More!.*

This book contains proven steps and strategies on how to use superfoods to achieve the best health. Superfoods have a tons of benefits in the body. Metabolism is increased and the body is detoxified, which improves organ functioning. They also can greatly help with weight loss and reduce inflammation, among many other amazing benefits!

In this book you will learn much more about these superfoods, and also how you can create healthy meals out of these foods!

Thanks again for purchasing this book, I hope you enjoy it!

Chapter 1: What Are Superfoods And How Can They Help You?

Superfoods are foods that have been informally named for their multiple and wide ranging health benefits. These are foods that are packed with nutrients that have very potent effects on the body.

These foods are mostly plant-based. However, some fish and dairy are also included in this food group. Superfoods are so-named because they are nutritionally dense. That is, there have high levels of vitamins and minerals that support health. In addition to these, they are also packed with special compounds. They have provide rich supplies of antioxidants that rid the body of free radicals and toxins, detoxify the liver and other organs, and protects tissues from damage. They also have compounds that have anticancer properties.

Superfoods are also rich in trace elements that support several bodily functions. They accelerate certain enzyme actions to boost health.

These foods also have an abundance of compounds that have potent anti-cancer properties. They protect the body from damage that can trigger the development of cancer. They also strengthen the immune system to fight off cancer-causing compounds and infections.

Other benefits from superfoods include strengthening the tissues. They also improve blood flow to the tissues. Blood brings oxygen and nutrients to the cells. t also takes cell debris and wastes out of the tissues and to the excretory organs. Good blood flow means good efficient exchange of nutrients and wastes. This way, the body gets to function more efficiently.

Superfoods also strengthen the digestive system. This way, food is better digested, absorbed ad delivered to the different tissues.

There are also a lot more benefits from the many compounds in the different superfoods. Just take care to consume in moderation. Some superfoods include fruits that have sugar and fats in them. Overconsumption can cause imbalance, despite the many health benefits.

Thanks for Previewing My Exciting Book Entitled:

"Superfoods: Ultimate Superfoods Health And Diet Detox Guide! - Increase Metabolism, Natural Beauty And Health With 50 Powerful Natural Remedies And Recipes For Anti-Aging, Fat Loss, And More!"

To purchase this book, simply go to the Amazon Kindle store and simply search:

"SUPERFOODS"

Then just scroll down until you see my book. You will know it is mine because you will see my name "Sarah Brooks" underneath the title.

Alternatively, you can visit my author page on Amazon to see this book and other work I have done. Thanks so much, and please don't forget your free bonuses.

DON'T LEAVE YET! - CHECK OUT YOUR FREE BONUSES BELOW!

Free Bonus Offer: Get Free Access To The www.LiveFitVIP.com VIP Newsletter!

Once you enter your email address you will immediately get free access to this awesome newsletter!

But wait, right now if you join now for free you will also get free access to the "The 7 Keys To Body Transformation" free EBook!

To claim both your FREE VIP NEWSLETTER MEMBERSHIP and your FREE BONUS EBook on THE 7 KEYS TO BODY TRANSFORMATION!

Just Go To:

www.liveFitVIP.com

www.ingramcontent.com/pod-product-compliance
Lightning Source LLC
Chambersburg PA
CBHW070939290526
45795CB00003B/1071